Laura Corn

101 Nights of Grrrreat Sex

Secret Sealed

Seductions for

Fun Loving

Couples

PARK AVENUE PUBLISHERS

DISCLAIMER
PLEASE READ BEFORE PROCEEDING

This book is sold with the understanding that it is intended solely for the use of informed, consenting, and hopefully monogamous adults who want to rejuvenate, enliven and sustain a great sexual relationship. The author is not a medical doctor or therapist. She has, however, studied this subject intensely for the past 8 years and is the best-selling author of five books in this genre. Almost every recipe in this book has been recommended by leading sexual therapists.

The reader is cautioned that following the suggestions and scenarios contained herein is strictly voluntary and at the readers risk and discretion. Also, this book talks about sex acts which are illegal in some states. Know your state's law about sex and break them at your own risk. The positions and products mentioned in the book are safe and satisfying for the majority of adult women and men, every individual is unique and you should not employ any position or product which is not suitable to your physical or sexual limitations.

Neither the author, publisher or distributor endorses any specific product or assumes any product liability for any product mentioned in this book. The choices and responsibility for any consequences which may result from the use of any product or following any suggestion or scenario herein belong to the reader.

The author and Park Avenue Publishers, Inc., shall have neither liability nor responsibility to any person or entity with regard to any losses or damage caused or alleged to be caused, either directly or indirectly, by the information contained in this book.

If you do not wish to be bound by the above understanding, you may return the book intact to Park Avenue Publishers, Inc., PO Box 20010, Oklahoma City, OK 73156, for a full refund of the purchase price of the book.

Cover Design Concept by Ron Larson

ACKNOWLEDGEMENTS

I am deeply indebted to a host of people who made this book possible. I have been especially fortunate to have so many wonderful teachers, friends and business associates. To each of them, I extend my heartfelt gratitude:

First and foremost, to the women and men in radio all across this continent, the brightest, funniest, hardest working people in creation, who provided the forum and granted me the audience which made my first book, "237 Intimate Questions Every Woman Should Ask A Man", a best-seller while enabling me to gather the knowledge and material for "101 Nights of Grrreat Sex."

To Joann Rossi, my friend, counselor, and confidante, whose contribution to both the concept and content of the book is priceless and whom I cannot thank enough for her loyalty, patience and dedication.

To Marty Bishop, DJ extraordinaire, whose fertile imagination and flair permeates this book and for whom I cannot find words eloquent enough to express my gratitude for his inestimable assistance and contribution.

To Bill Wright, my forever friend and shepherd, for his continuing support, faith and love through all the ups and downs. You love unconditionally and motivate me to achieve the impossible. No one has had more positive influence on me in my life.

To Michael Hutchinson, friend and mentor for his encouragement, for championing this project and for his advice and guidance into the wonderful world of direct response.

To J.P. my best friend in the whole wide world. Thank you for sharing this journey with me. Your love, encouragement and understanding inspires me everyday.

And last, but not least I am grateful to Larry Paregis, Tim Daze, Paul Nugas, Tracy & Donald Sonck, Kimberly Bennett, Marcella Gallagher, Bill Stamps, John & Cass Corn, Linda Seto, Jay Corn, Casandria & Dorothy Moore, and Terry.

And, to all the people who bought my books, responded to me on the air, stood in line for hours for a personal word with me, endured my probing interviews and opened up their hearts, minds and souls to provide me with the most essential ingredient in this book; their desires, needs and experiences.

TABLE OF CONTENTS

INTRODUCTION TO *GRRREAT* SEX!

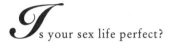s your sex life perfect?

Are you totally thrilled, aroused, and satisfied after every erotic encounter? Is your life behind the bedroom door absolutely, completely, overwhelmingly fulfilling?

Then put this book down!!

Somebody else needs it more than you.

Most of us, in fact, find it all too easy to let *life* get in the way of love. Jobs and bills and chores and kids all conspire to push intimacy to the bottom of our list of priorities. If we can make any private time at all for each other, it's only when we're tired and distracted. The same old moves, the same old positions, and after a while sex gets, well —

Boring. Boooorr-ring.

In survey after survey, ho-hum sex is the number one complaint of couples across the country. And it doesn't have to be that way.

Because this book guarantees grrreat sex. 101 nights of it, just like the title says!

That's every week, twice a week, for one full year. Now, I know that's a lot to ask from one little book! But I promise you that it works. Here's how —

Every week, you and your partner flip through it, discussing the titles that catch your eye. This can be a real blast — it's a little like window-shopping for sex! Each of you then tears a page from the book, and in that one special moment, you've made a serious commitment to each other. You've created a new kind of bond between yourselves.

By removing a page right in front of you, your lover has just given a promise that, no matter what, *you are going to be seduced* in a fresh, exciting, original, and highly erotic manner. Sometime during the week, *your sensual pleasure* will be the only focus. You, of course, are making the same promise in return.

And neither of you has any idea what the other is planning! The pages are sealed, in fact, and you have to read yours in private. Each contains one complete seduction, written out step by delicious, detailed step. Some of them are simple, and fast, and fun — "quickies" designed to startle and delight your lover. If you've ever felt like sex was getting too darned predictable, just wait'll you get to Seduction Number... well, I think I'll keep that a secret for now, too.

On the other hand, some of these scenarios require a bit of planning. You might spend hours setting it up just right, and the end result will be absolutely unforgettable. There is nothing in the world quite so thrilling as the thought that someone went to a whole lot of effort to make you feel special. And best of all — *you get all the credit!* Remember, these recipes for love are a secret, and your bedmate will never know which ideas came from this book...and which were fueled by your own steamy and slightly naughty imagination.

You'll eventually notice some common threads linking these seductions, and here's one of the most important — almost all of them ask you do something to *tease your lover*. Often it's just a hint; the tiniest little clue left lying about early in the week to tantalize your bedmate, to remind your partner of the surprise in store. Now, if you find a seduction that's not exactly your cup of tea, feel free to change it. I'll bet you can come up with something that suits you even better! But please — please! — *keep that element of anticipation*. It's the heart and soul of this book. That sense of expectancy is more than just spice in the sauce. It's what elevates sex from mundane to magnificent. It transforms intercourse from an athletic event into one of the mysteries of the universe. It makes you feel like a kid again!

And speaking of kids — I know what you're thinking. They might be the light of your life and your hope for the future...but the little devils can certainly put a damper on the ol' libido, can't they? Well, for every parent who tells me they couldn't use this book because there's just not enough time — *and no privacy, for crying out loud!* — I have three things to say.

First, intimacy is more than just fun and games. It heals us and sustains us and renews our deepest feelings for each other — *make it a priority*. Besides, you've got almost a week to pull this off!

Second, isn't it important to teach by example? Show your children that playfulness and sensuality is an important part of a loving, adult relationship. If your kids see Mom and Dad laughing and touching and writing love-notes and chasing each other around the house for a kiss, then that's the kind of grown-ups they'll learn to be...and the world will be a better place for it.

And third, if you really are pressed for time and can only follow through on, say, just one seduction each week — then this book will last you *two* whole years. What a deal!

And believe me, whether you have kids or not, once you make this a weekly practice, you'll *find* the time to carry it out. You'll come to covet these special moments together. That's because these seductions were created to give each of you *exactly what you're looking for* — that is, if you're anything like the thousands of people I've talked to over the years!

On hundreds of radio shows across the country, and all during the time I was preparing my first book, *237 Intimate Questions Every Woman Should Ask A Man,* I heard what men and women want in the bedroom. We want to know how to turn our mates on. We want them to know what turns *us* on. We'd like more variety...more foreplay...more surprises...more interest...new tricks...and once in a while, somebody *else* should do all the work! And that's what gave me the idea for this book:

Fifty seductions written for *his eyes only,* spelling out exactly how to get her attention, how to make her laugh, how to make her want you — and how to bring her to new heights of passion. Fifty seductions written for *her eyes only,* filled with clever and fun ways to spark his interest, each with an unusual twist or *advanced sexual technique* designed to fan that spark into a white-hot flame. And finally, one very special seduction to be read by both of you. Number 101 is a sort of graduation exercise for my newest Masters of The Erotic Arts — save this one for last!

And from start to finish, every single one of them is designed to make your mate feel like a million bucks. No halfhearted measures in this book! Every week, when it's your turn to turn on, you'll flirt and tease. You'll arouse. You'll build anticipation. You'll use new techniques. Just think of the fun you'll have when you bring your lover to a huge, gigantic, bedshaking, weak-at-the-knees, leave-'em-gasping, ohmigodimcomingrightnow ORGASM!!! And isn't it nice to know that you're guaranteed the same treatment in return?

There's more to *101 Nights Of Grrreat Sex* than, well, great sex. There's a wealth of wisdom and knowledge packed in here, too. On the page opposite each seduction you'll find terrific and useful sexual advice culled from fifty-four of the best-selling books in the field. In fact, almost every recipe in here has been recommended by doctors and therapists who are recognized as experts in human sexuality.

Most of these seductions also include something I like to call *frostings...* special bedroom skills that can bring you closer to your sexual peak and keep you there longer. And you can use them to drive your sweetie absolutely crazy!

But instead of simply explaining new techniques, this book incorporates them into each fun, erotic episode. This is not like some new diet, where you're expected to simply change your lifestyle overnight. *Here, you'll learn by doing* — slowly, gradually, month-by-month. And because you're doing it often — every week, remember, for a whole year — you'll actually turn interesting, exhilarating, unpredictable sex into a *habit,* and not just a special event.

I must confess that many of the ideas in this book are not originally mine. They were dreamed up by ordinary people from all over the country — regular folks who use these techniques to bring sexual excitement back into a mature relationship. I can't close this introduction without a word of thanks for their contribution to the book.

There are too many to list, and I don't even know all their names, but I'm sure they'll recognize their little tricks scattered throughout these pages! They managed to ride through the flood of phone calls we get on the radio and tell us the secrets to long term happiness in a relationship. They shared with us their knack for keeping sex fun and interesting months, years, and even decades into a partnership. They taught us about the importance of *comfort* — both in and out of our clothes.

And they helped me develop the formula for this book. The anticipation of an erotic encounter, plus the surprises you spring on your love, plus the excitement of the seduction itself, plus the thrill of trying new things with your lover — it all adds up to truly *Great Sex.* Don't just read about it. Do it! And thank me later.

Laura Corn

Santa Monica, California
January 2000

Now — some final notes before you start your big adventure —

Hygiene. It's critical! I can't tell you how many men and women have told me they've lost interest in sex because their partner has some personal grooming flaws. Think of it this way — as you go through this book, your love is going to kiss and nibble and lick and suck various parts of you, a *lot!* You're going to do the same. Neither of you wants any, um, unpleasant surprises, and you sure don't want to give a reason not to do it again! Fresh breath, clean teeth, shampooed hair, and scrubbed skin — it's the uniform you put on *before* the game of love.

Money. Most of these seductions cost nothing at all. But for those that do, I've included little icons on the title pages to give you an idea of what to expect.

No $ at all means it's free, or under ten dollars.

$	means 10 to 25 dollars.
$$	means 30 to 60 dollars.
$$$	means 65 to 100 dollars.
☆	means over a hundred dollars.

Yes, there are even a couple that cost a lot — if your budget permits, the sky's the limit. And yes, I think you *should* plan one or two seductions every year where you pull out all the stops! Anniversaries, Birthdays, Valentine's Day, etc...What you're buying are memories that will last a lifetime.

The rest of the icons. The car means you're going somewhere. The sun means you need nice weather. The fork-and-spoon indicates a meal is involved.

Props. Lots of these seductions encourage you to buy extra little items to dress up the event. Most are inexpensive and easy to find, and to help you locate any that aren't available in your town, I've included a list of mail-order catalogues in the back of the book. Don't just ignore these special ingredients! It's extra touches like these that convince your sweetheart you really mean it. If you can't find what I've suggested, *substitute*. Use your imagination. It really is the effort that counts.

How to do it. Set aside one evening per week to look through the book. Sunday night is a good idea...you're relaxed, and you've got almost a whole week to plan the details of your seduction. Both of you get to pick one page, and then tear it out of the book. There's no turning back now! Your partner saw you do it, and is now expecting you to follow through. And of course, you'll be getting an erotic surprise sometime this week, too. Delicious idea, isn't it? The days will fly by!

Getting seduced. It may take a lot of nerve for your love to try some of these recipes, especially the ones that call for, um, bold behavior. So play along! Be encouraging. You will *not* regret it.

The Law. Hey, nothing in here is illegal. I think.

Laura Corn, I just CAN'T do that! Yes, you can. Sooner or later, especially if you're a shy person, chances are you'll come across a seduction that seems too wild or too extravagant or simply too much for you. I say — just do it! Do it do it do it! Almost a million other couples have already, so please give it a try. Your partner might be thrilled. you might learn to love something new. And if you can't, well, at least don't give up on your promise to your mate. Pull out another seduction ... or make up one of your own! The important thing is to make your partner's pleasure a top priority at least once a week.

Did I mention GRRREAT sex? That is, of course, only if you finish this introduction, grab your partner, and start tearing out pages. Go on — start right now. I'm done.

You, on the other hand, are just beginning. It's a one-year course in the ancient art of seduction, and when you're done, you'll have one tattered, empty book cover....

And a lot of *grrreat* memories.

Enjoy!

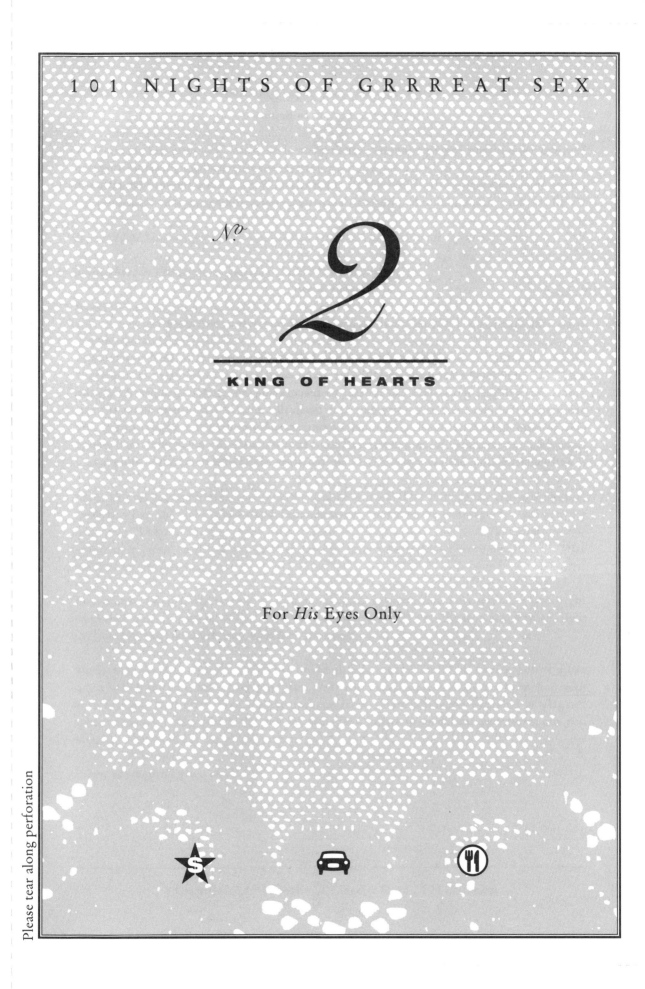

N.º

2

KING OF HEARTS

For *His* Eyes Only

No.

3

UP AGAINST THE WALL

For *His* Eyes Only

$

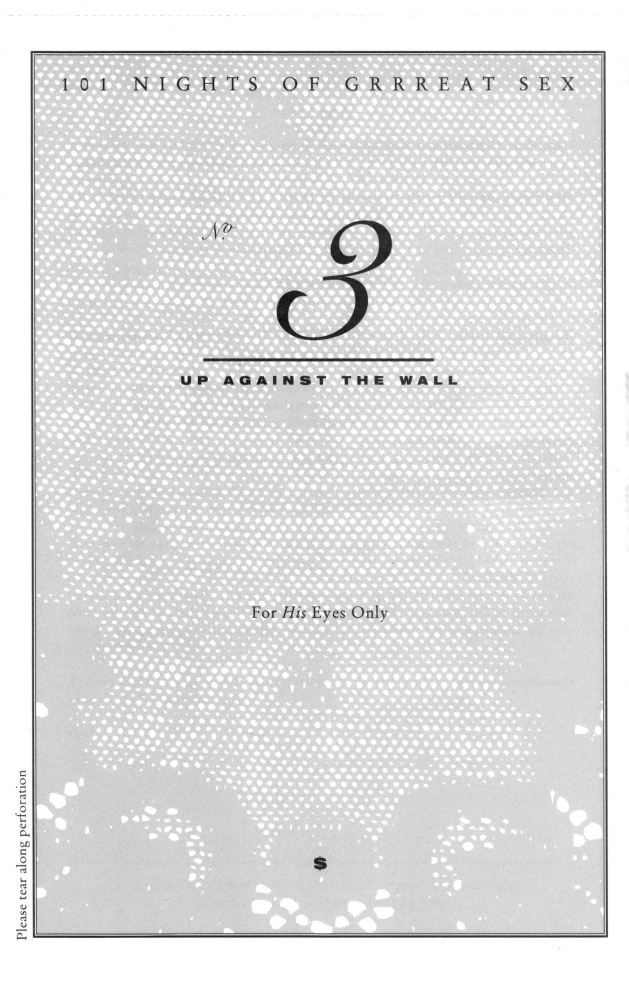

N.º

4

BURIED TREASURE

For *Her* Eyes Only

$

N.º

5

THE VELVET TONGUE

For *Her* Eyes Only

N.º

6

OBSTACLE COURSE

For *His* Eyes Only

N.º **7**

DANGEROUS WHEN WET

For *His* Eyes Only

№ **8**

THAT WILL BE THREE HUNDRED DOLLARS, PLEASE

For *Her* Eyes Only

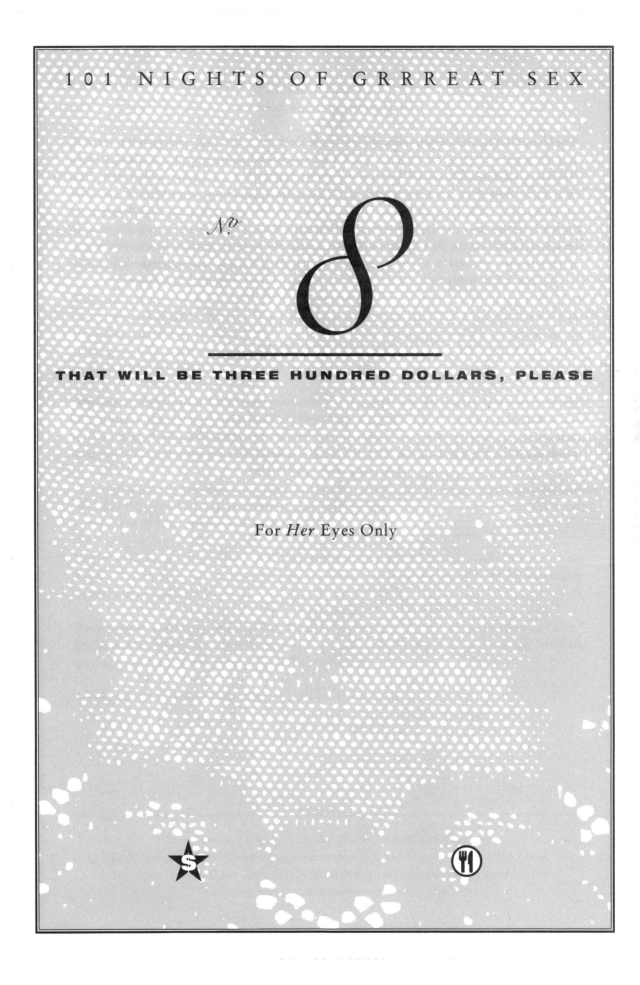

N.º

9

UNDER THE HOOD, COWBOY

For *His* Eyes Only

N.º

10

LINGERIE PARFAIT

For *Her* Eyes Only

$

N.º

11

ANGEL WITH A LARIAT

For *Her* Eyes Only

N.º

12

SOMEBODY STOP ME!

For *His* Eyes Only

$$

N.º

13

BEAT AROUND THE BUSH

For *Her* Eyes Only

$ ☀ 🚗

№ *14*

FIRE DOWN BELOW

For *His* Eyes Only

N°

15

THE LAURA CORN CHALLENGE

For *Her* Eyes Only

N.o

16

THE GEE! STROKE

For *His* Eyes Only

$

N⁰ **17**

TOOL TIME

For *His* Eyes Only

$

N°

18

THE THRILL OF THE CHASE

For *Her* Eyes Only

N^o *19*

SCHWING!

For *Her* Eyes Only

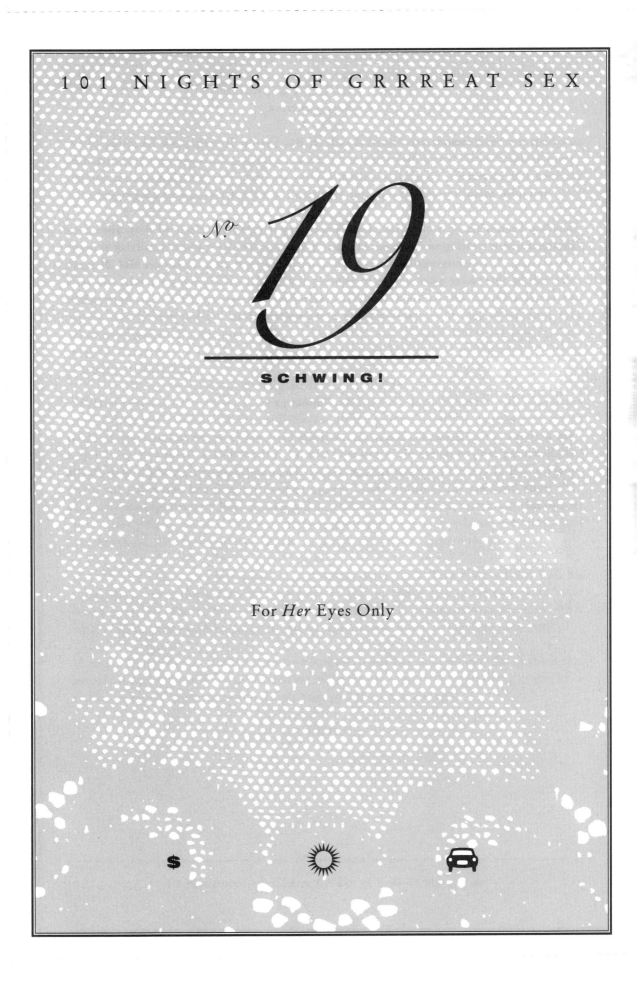

N.o

20

DOWN AND DIRTY

For *Her* Eyes Only

N.º

21

WILD CARD

For *Her* Eyes Only

N.º

23

THE SECRET DESSERT

For *Her* Eyes Only

$$ 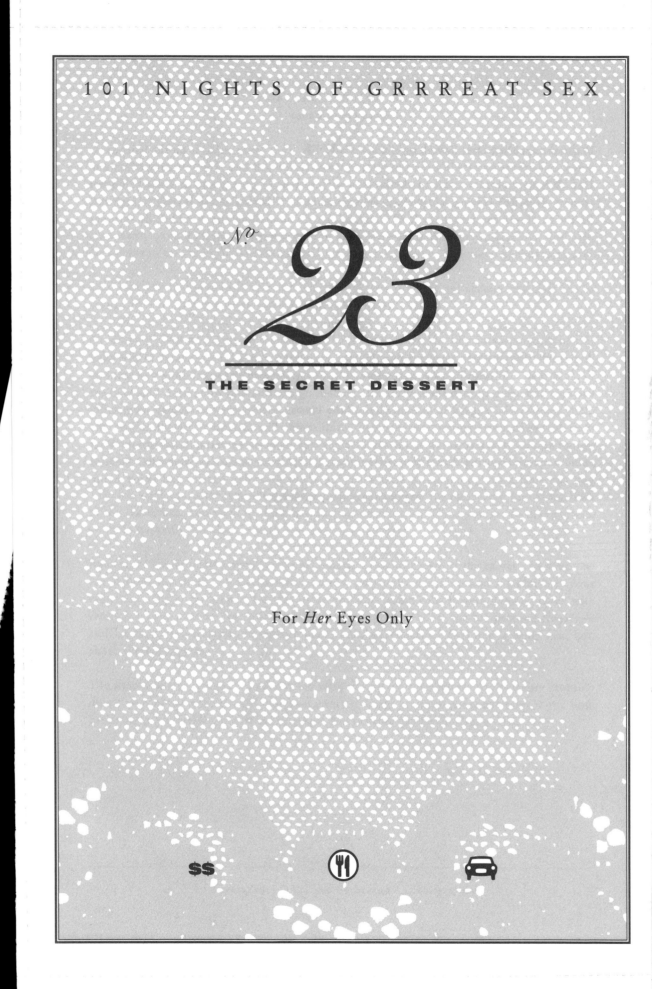 🍴 🚗

N.º 24

HONEY BREASTS & CREAMY THIGHS

For *His* Eyes Only

N.º

25

FINGER LICKIN' GOOD

For *His* Eyes Only

$

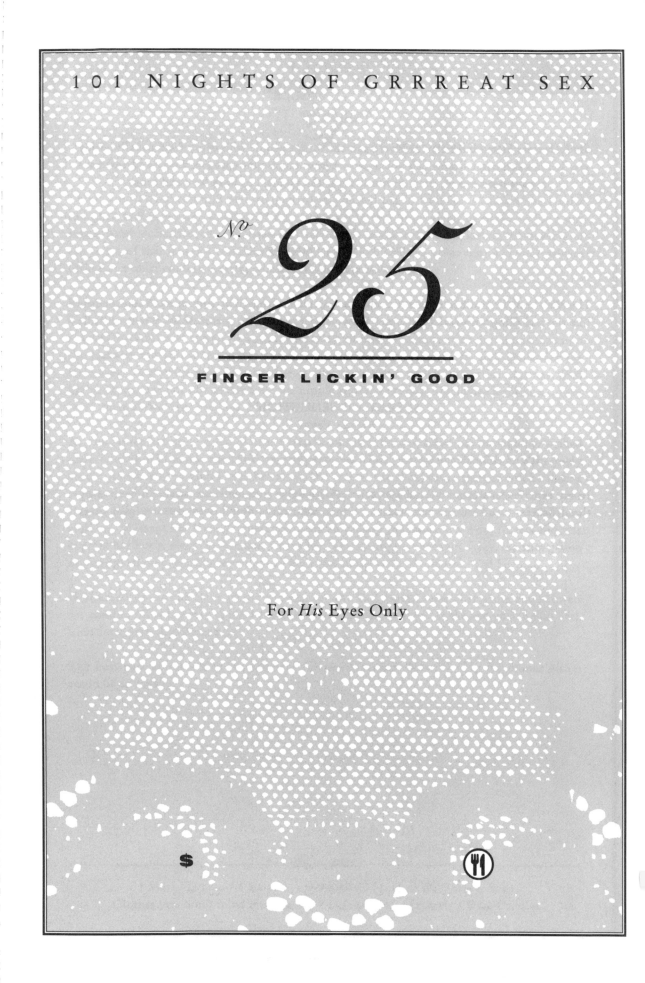

N.º **27**

TAKEN BY SURPRISE

For *His* Eyes Only

N.º **28**

A QUIET ECSTASY

For *Her* Eyes Only

N° 29

JONI'S BUTTERFLY

For *His* Eyes Only

$

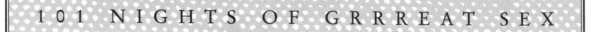

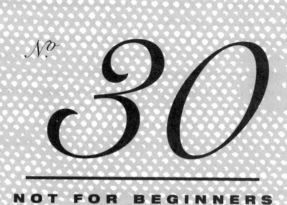

NOT FOR BEGINNERS

For *Her* Eyes Only

N.º 31

THE ONE HOUR ORGASM

For *Her* Eyes Only

N.º

32

WAVES OF DESIRE

For *His* Eyes Only

$

N.º

33

IT'S NOT ON THE MENU

For *Her* Eyes Only

$$ 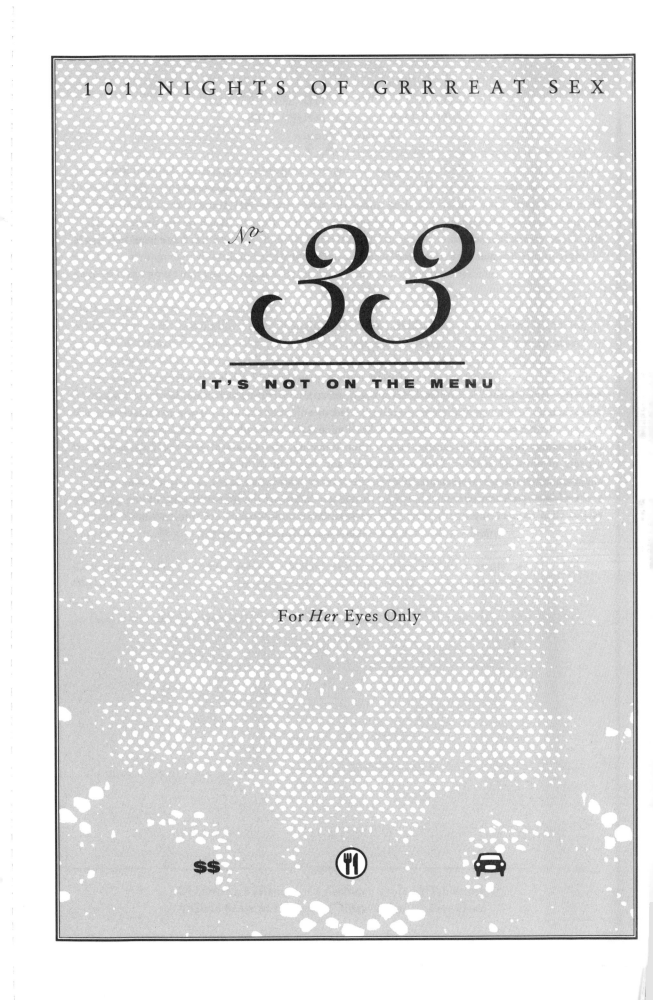 🚗

N.°

35

PLEASE FEED THE BEAR!

For *Her* Eyes Only

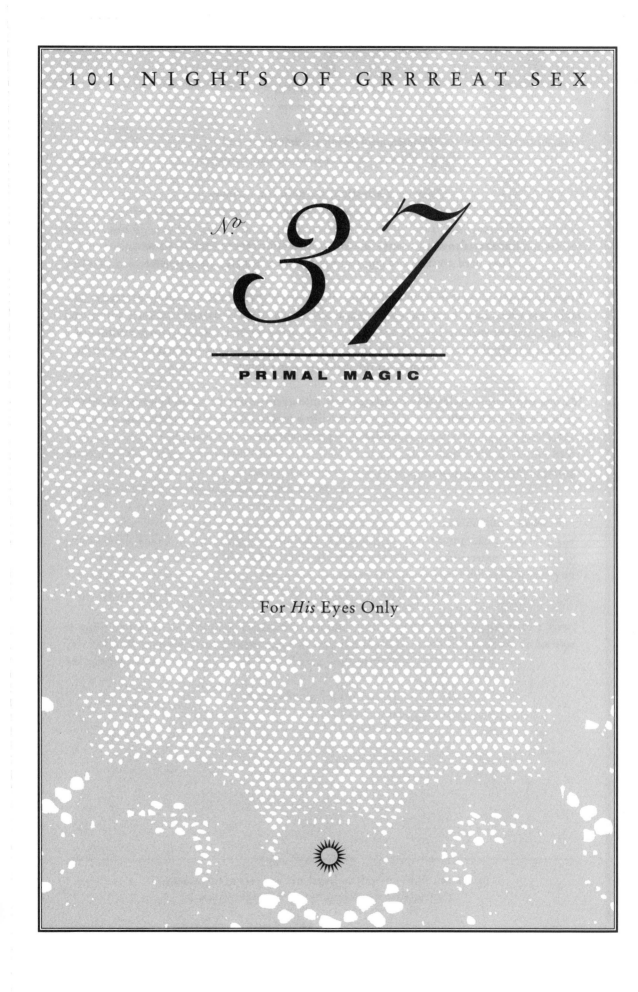

No. 37

___

PRIMAL MAGIC

For *His* Eyes Only

N° 38

___

THE EROTIC EQUATION

For *Her* Eyes Only

N.° **39**

WHERE NOBODY KNOWS YOUR NAME

For *His* Eyes Only

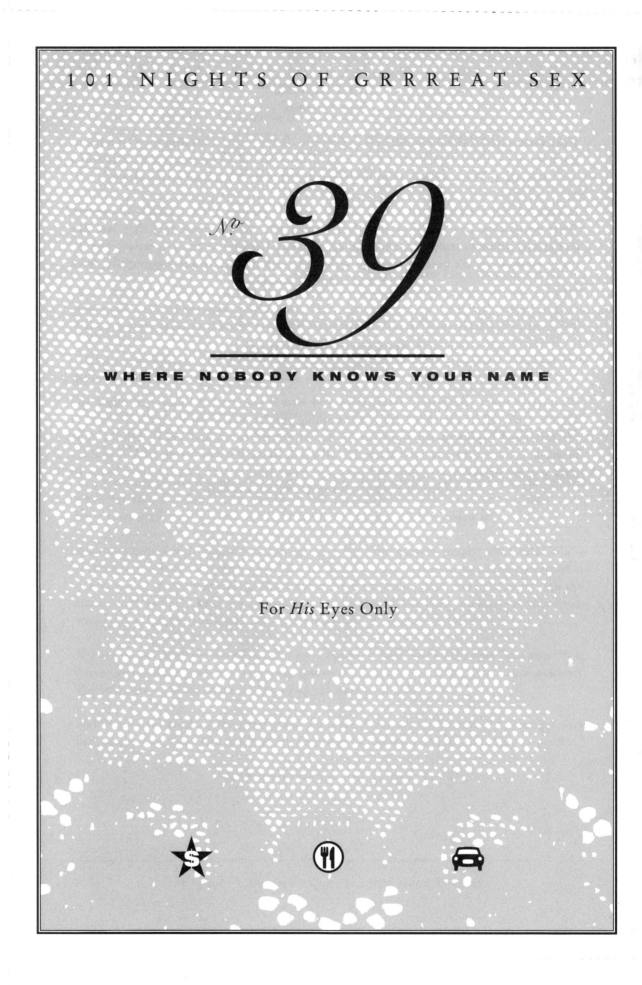

N.º **40**

MATING CALL

For *His* Eyes Only

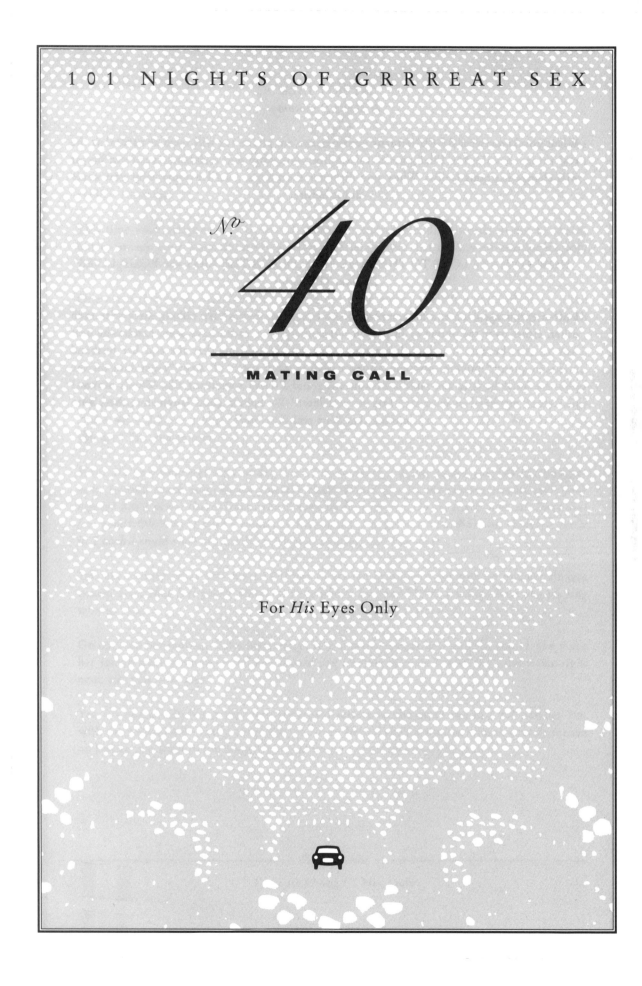

N.º **41**

SIXTY MINUTE MAN

For *His* Eyes Only

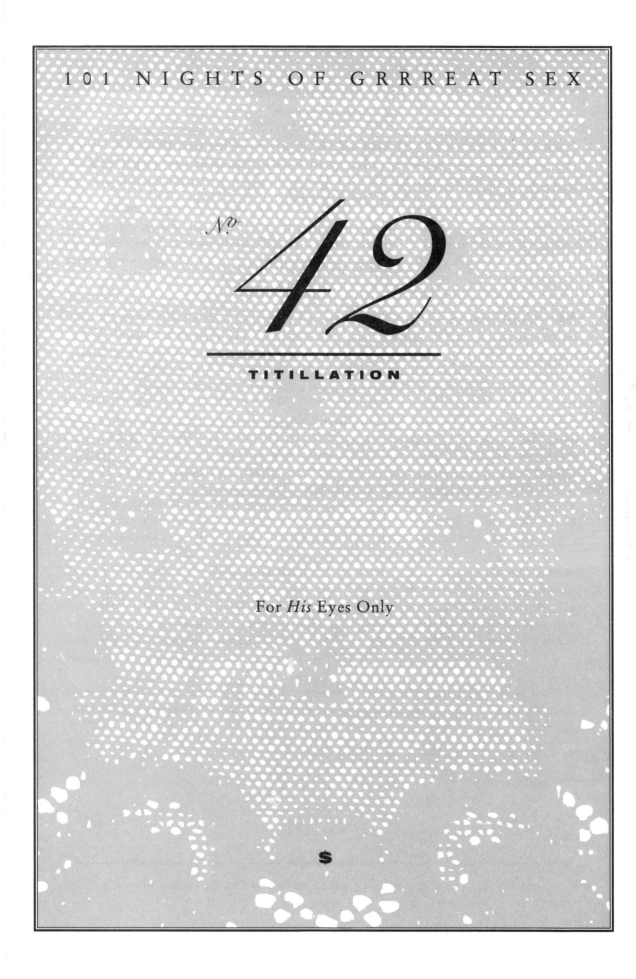

Nº 42

TITILLATION

For *His* Eyes Only

$

No. 43

LEAVE IT TO BEAVER

For *Her* Eyes Only

N° 44

HALFTIME SHENANIGANS

For *Her* Eyes Only

N.º

1

"I THINK I MADE HIS BACK FEEL BETTER"

For *Her* Eyes Only

Nº 45

SLAVETIME!

For *His* Eyes Only

N.º **46**

LE FEMME FATALE

For *Her* Eyes Only

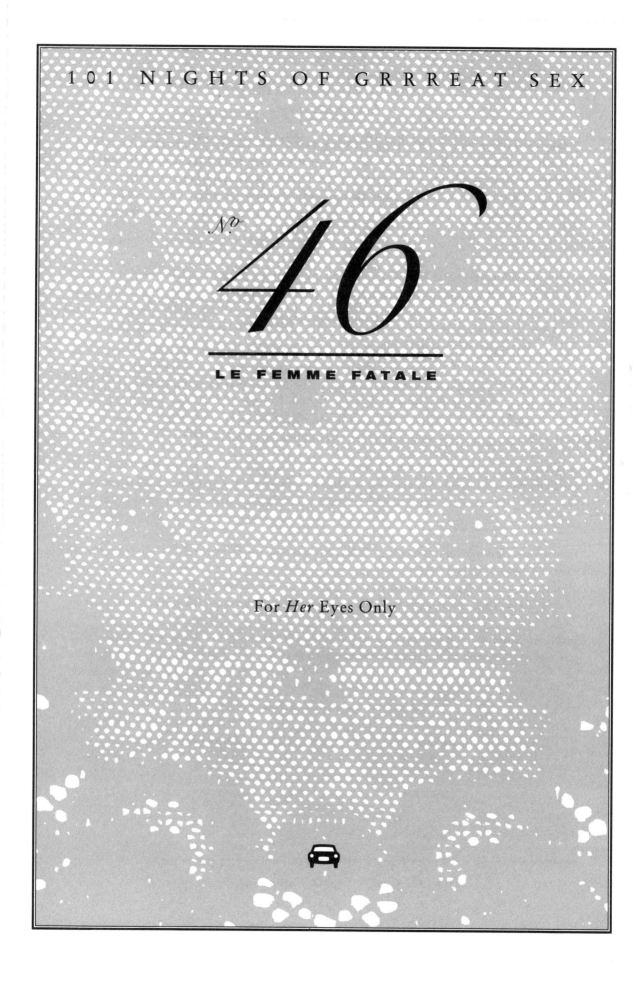

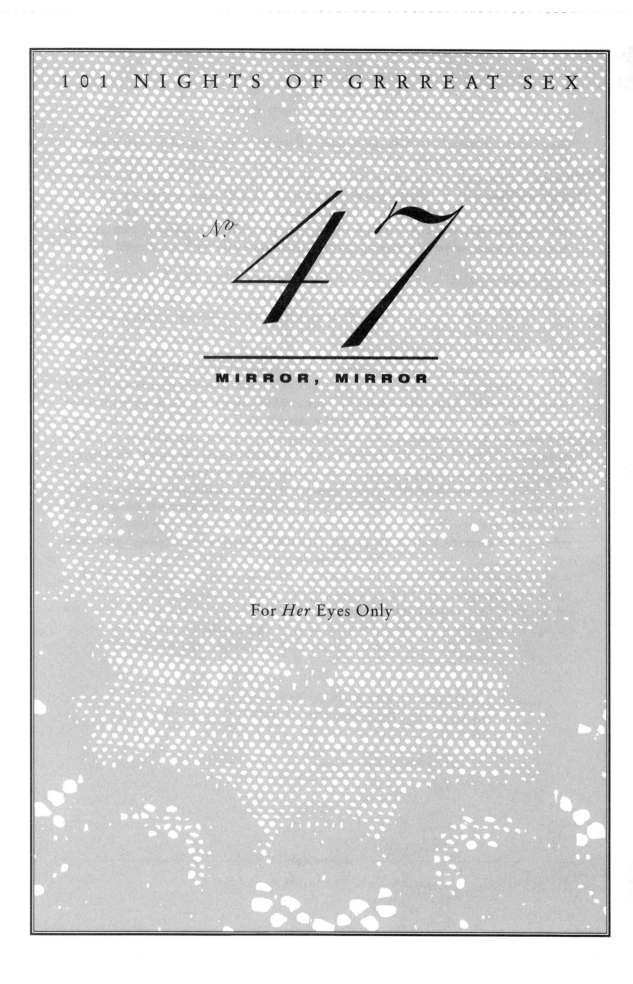

N.º 47

MIRROR, MIRROR

For *Her* Eyes Only

N.o 48

A SUDDEN GLIMPSE OF LACE

For *Her* Eyes Only

$

N.º 49

NIGHT MOVES

For *Her* Eyes Only

$$

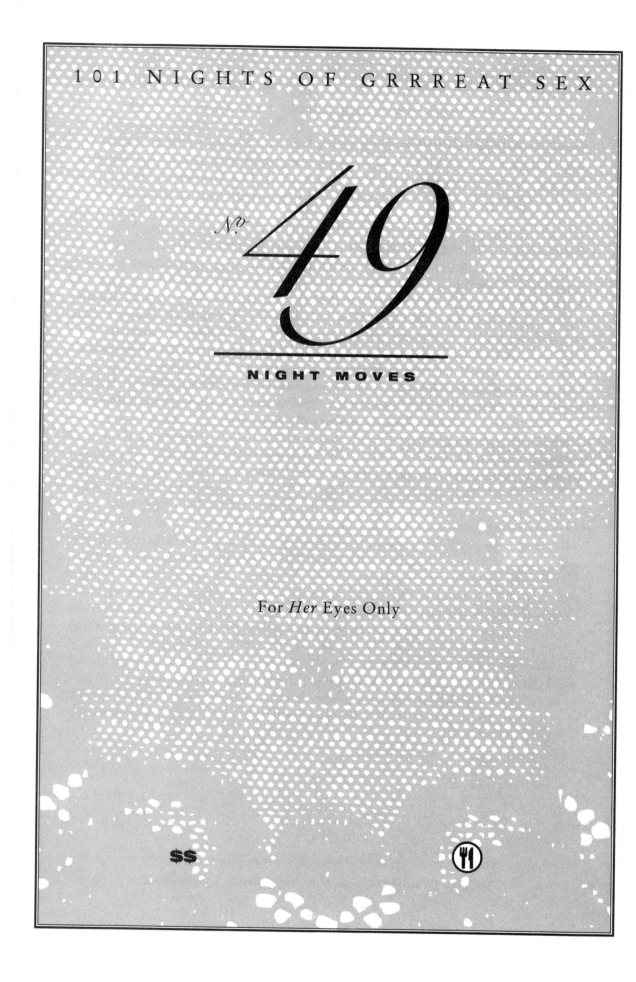

N^{o} **50**

SUBLIMINAL SEDUCER

For *His* Eyes Only

$$$ 🍽   🚗

N.º

51

RADIO PURR-DUCER

For *His* Eyes Only

N.º

52

MORNING GLORY

For *His* Eyes Only

No ## 53

ON TOP OF SUGAR MOUNTAIN

For *Her* Eyes Only

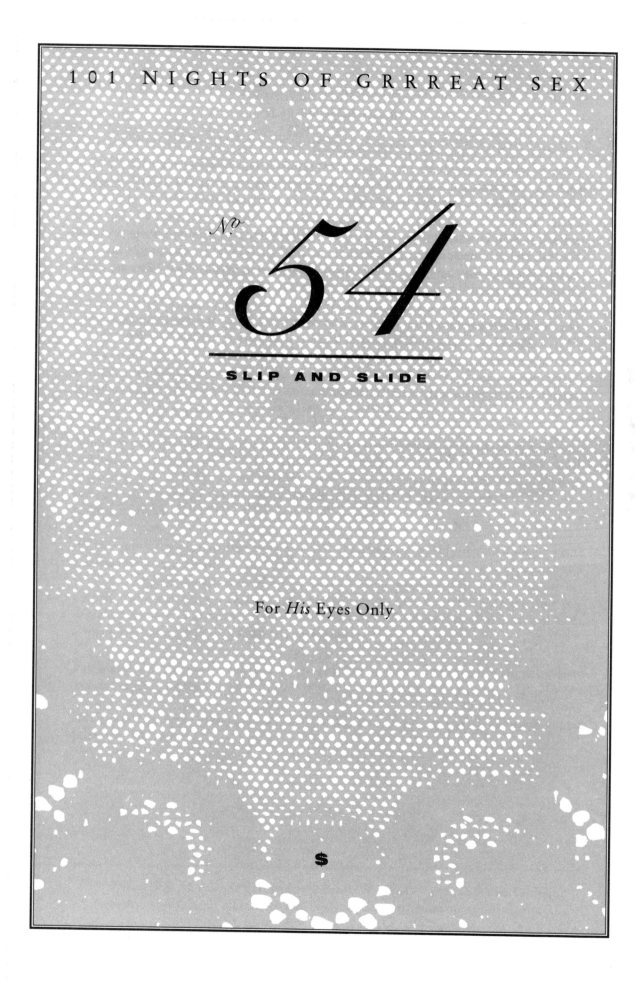

N.º

54

SLIP AND SLIDE

For *His* Eyes Only

$

№ 55

SWEET SURRENDER

For *Her* Eyes Only

$

N.º

56

THE PERFECT TOUCH

For *Her* Eyes Only

N.º **57**

TICKLED PINK

For His Eyes Only

$$

N.º

58

THE SENSUOUS SQUEEZE

For *Her* Eyes Only

$

N.º **59**

DELICIOUS DETOUR

For *Her* Eyes Only

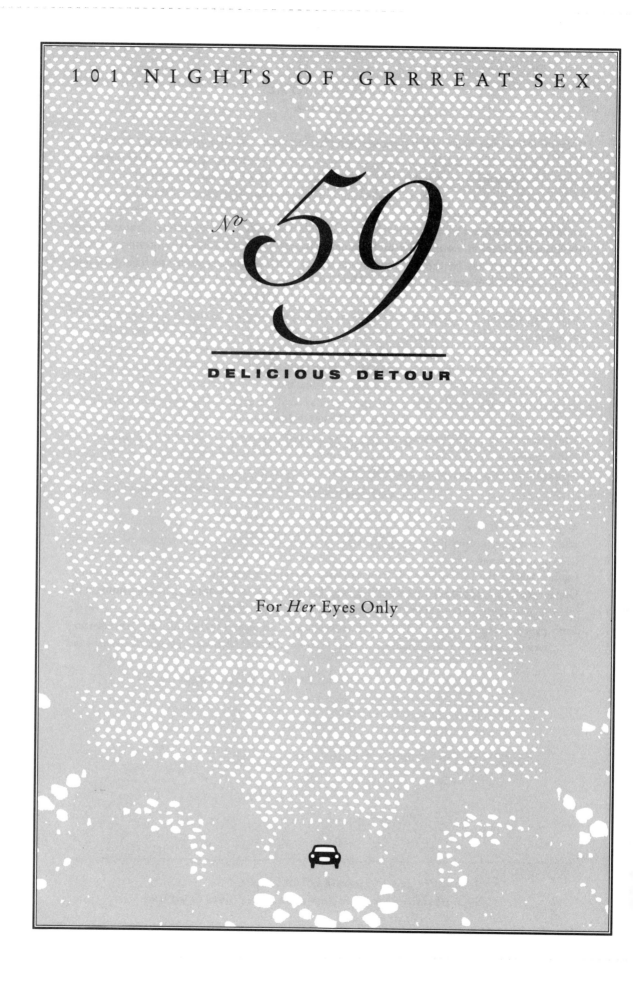

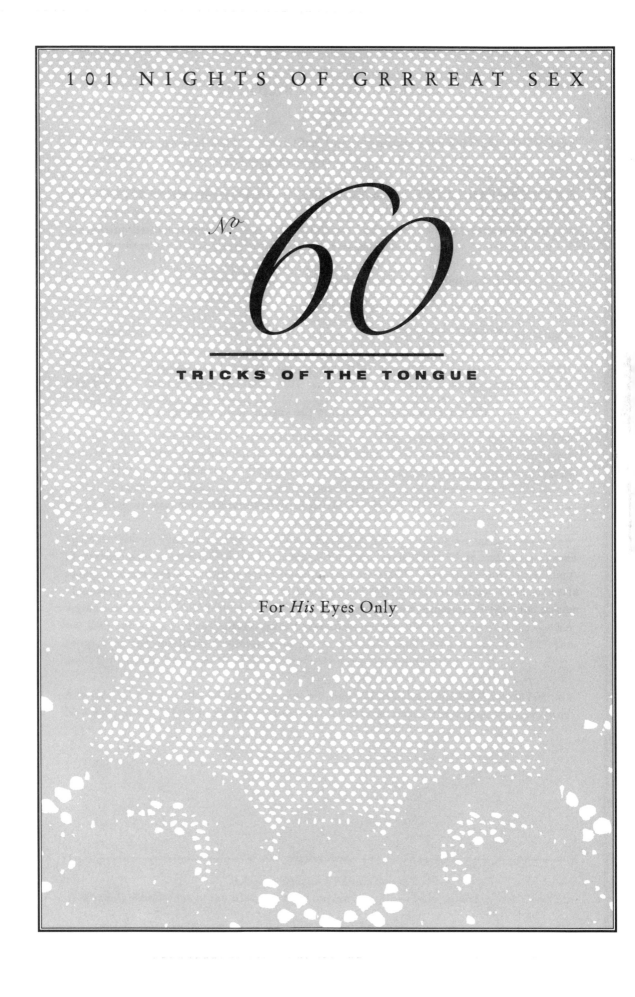

N.º

60

TRICKS OF THE TONGUE

For *His* Eyes Only

N^o *61*

SEVEN SINFUL FLAVORS

For *Her* Eyes Only

$

N.º

62

PENILINGUS

For *Her* Eyes Only

N^{o}

63

THE PIZZA MAN ALWAYS RINGS TWICE

For *His* Eyes Only

$

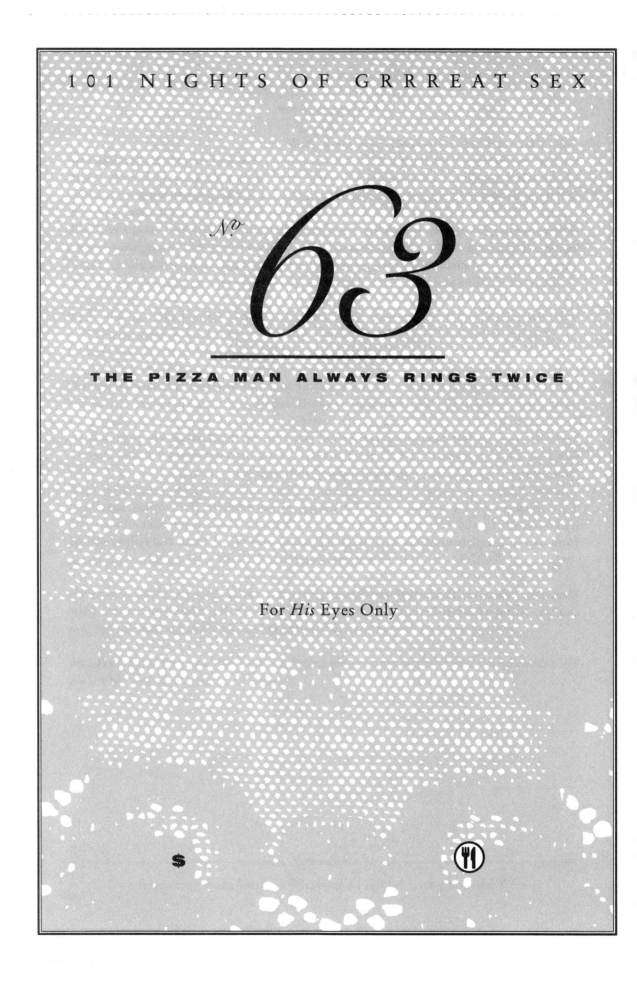

N.º **64**

FOUR LITTLE WIGGLY FINGERS

For *His* Eyes Only

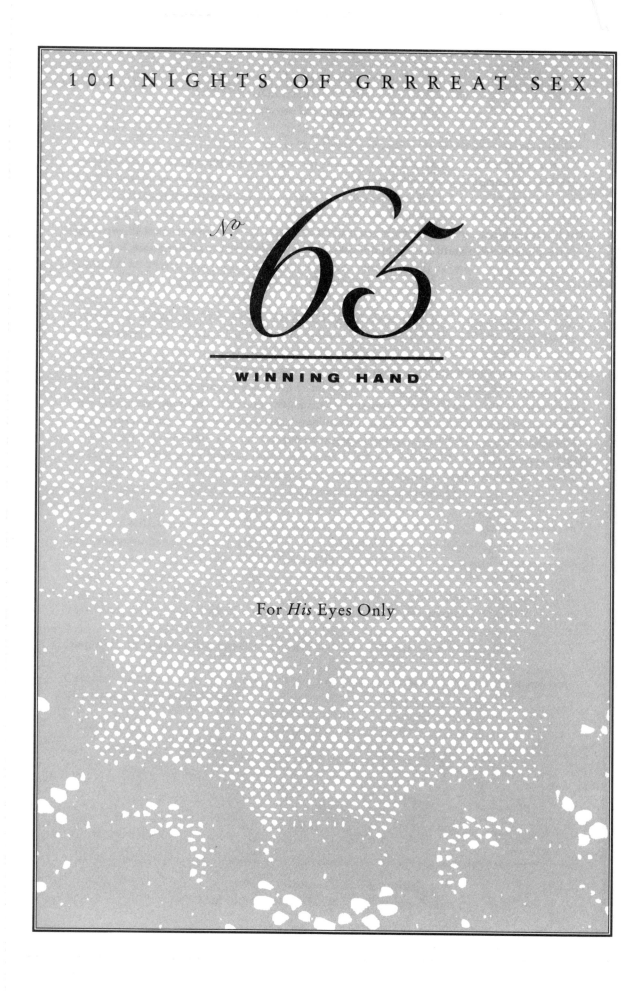

N.º

65

WINNING HAND

For *His* Eyes Only

N.º

66

THE FRENCH CONNECTION

For *His* Eyes Only

N.º 67

TENDER OUTLAW

For *His* Eyes Only

$

№ **68**

PUSS 'N BOOTS

For *Her* Eyes Only

$$

Nº **69**

THE CAT TECHNIQUE

For *His* Eyes Only

N⁰ 70

WET AND WILD

For *His* Eyes Only

$

N° 71

RED LIGHT DISTRICT

For *Her* Eyes Only

$$

$\mathcal{N}^o$ **72**

_____

CYBORGASM

For *Her* Eyes Only

$

N^o **73**

DOUBLE THE PLEASURE

For *Her* Eyes Only

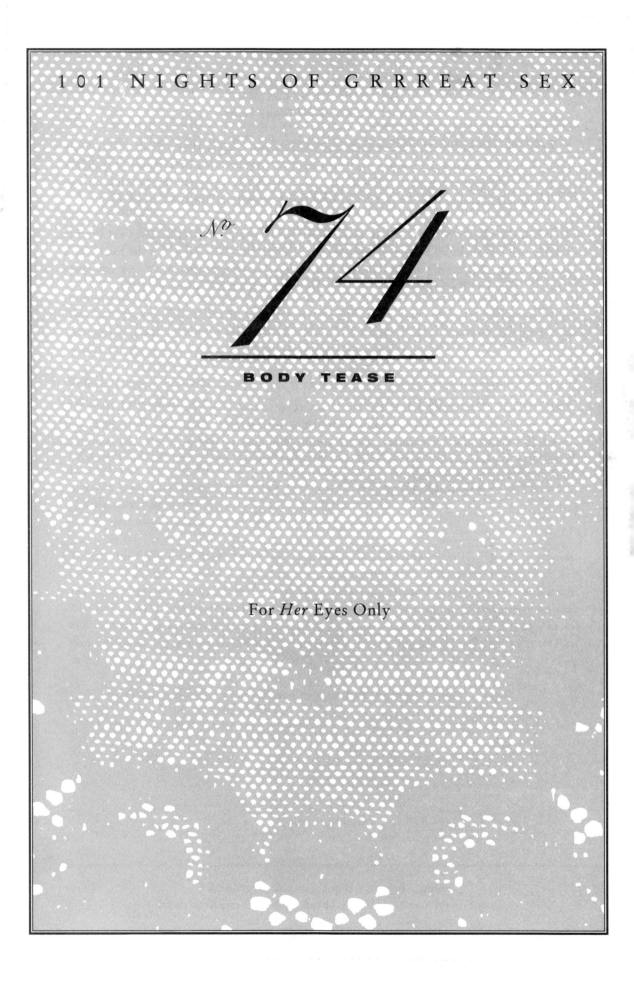

N.o 74

BODY TEASE

For *Her* Eyes Only

N° 75

THE KISS OF LEATHER

For *His* Eyes Only

$

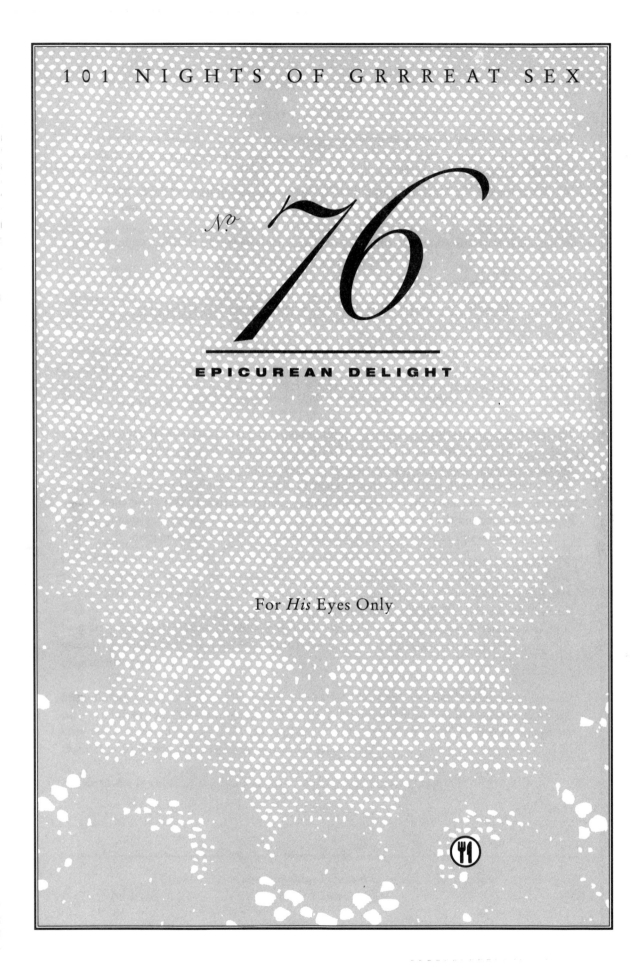

N.º 76

EPICUREAN DELIGHT

For *His* Eyes Only

N.º 77

WILD CARD

For *His* Eyes Only

N° 78

MUSTANG SALLY

For *Her* Eyes Only

ss · 🍴 · 🚗

N⁰ 79

MERCY!

For *His* Eyes Only

N.o 80

SEX IN A SHOE BOX

For *His* Eyes Only

N.º **81**

THE PLEASURE PRINCIPAL

For *Her* Eyes Only

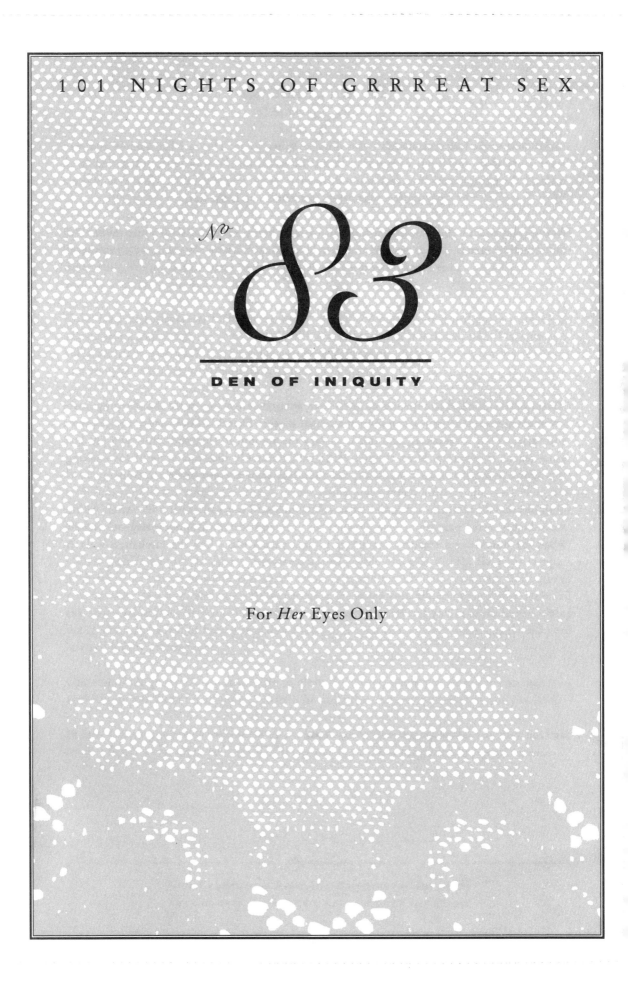

N.º

83

DEN OF INIQUITY

For *Her* Eyes Only

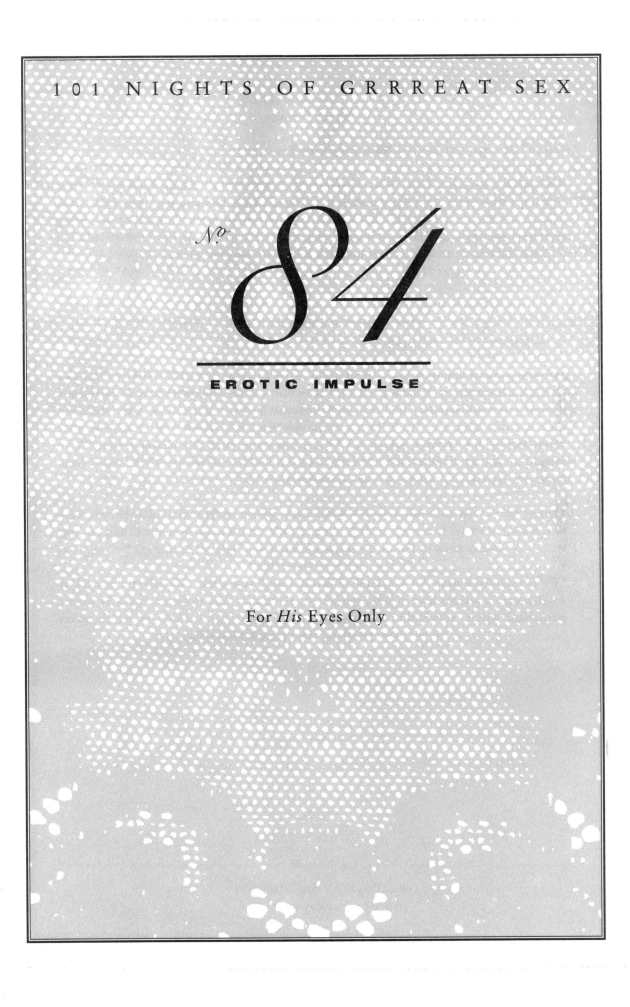

N° 84

EROTIC IMPULSE

For *His* Eyes Only

N.º 85

HOT LUNCH

For *Her* Eyes Only

$$ 🍴   🚗

№ **88**

PANDORA'S BOX

For *Her* Eyes Only

No. *89*

DOCTOR YES

For *His* Eyes Only

$

N.º *91*

THE BIG SCORE

For *His* Eyes Only

N^o

92

HIGH RENT RENDEZVOUS

For *His* Eyes Only

$$$

N.º

93

POINT OF NO RETURN

For *His* Eyes Only

$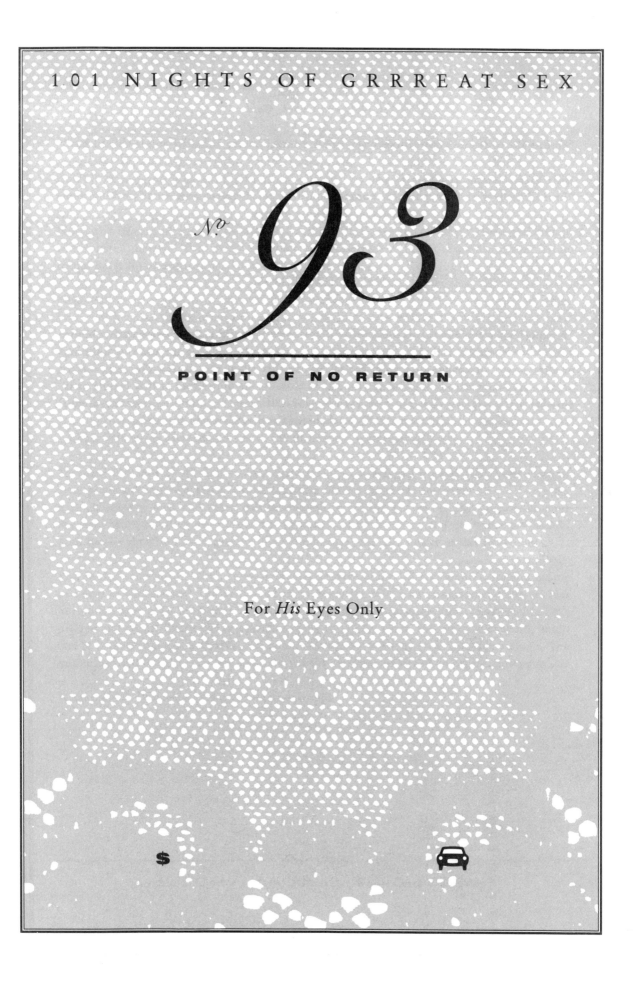

N.o **95**

THE SEXUAL LEXICON

For *Her* Eyes Only

$

N.º 96

JUST FOR THE FUN OF IT

For *Her* Eyes Only

$

№ **97**

THREE THUMBS UP!

For *Her* Eyes Only

$ 🚗

Nº **99**

BARELY LEGAL

For *His* Eyes Only

$$$

N^o *100*

GATES OF HEAVEN

For *Her* Eyes Only

$

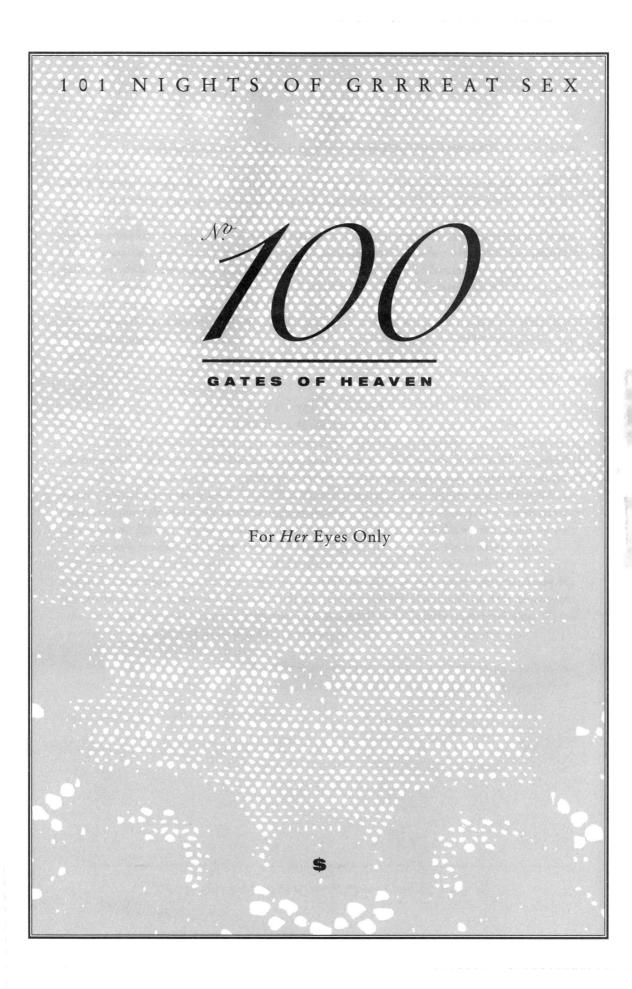

N.o

101

THE LAST SEDUCTION

For *Both* of You!

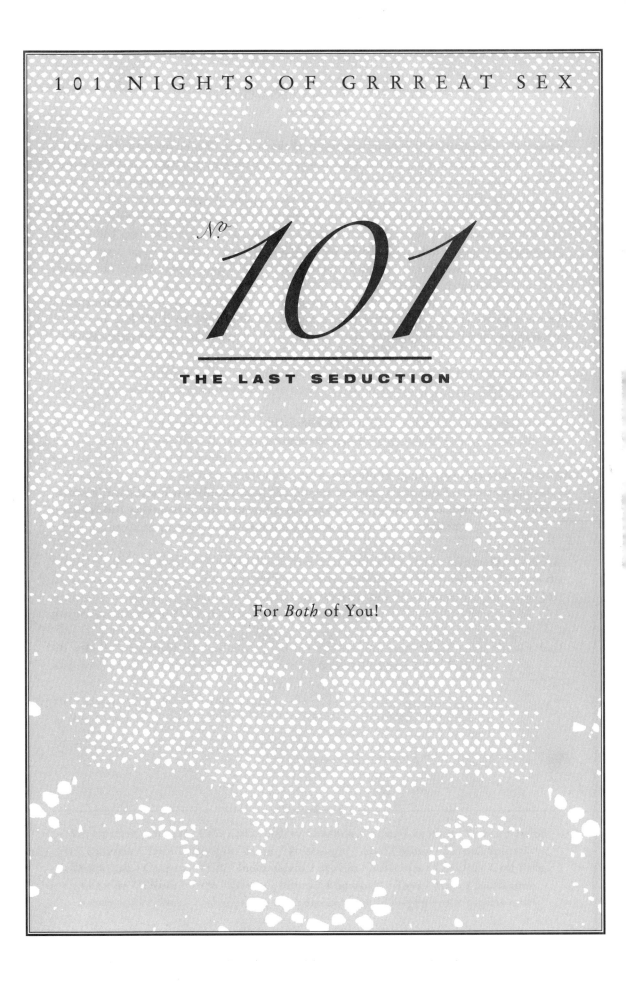

PERMISSIONS AND COPYRIGHT ACKNOWLEDGMENTS

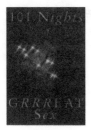
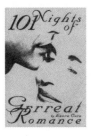
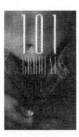
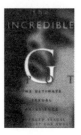

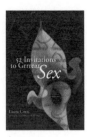

It All Begins With A Lick. . .52 Invitations to Great Sex!

Once a week-every week for an entire year *Grrreat Sex* is in the bag. (the mail bag!) Laura has created fifty-two brand new erotic adventures, each with a unique twist: an *invitation*, ready to be mailed to your lover. It's steamy but discreet; mysterious, yet perfectly clear. It means a night of heart-pounding, sheet splitting, toe-curling *sex* is on the way. . .
($29.95 + $4.95 shipping & handling)

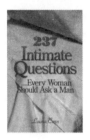

237 Intimate Questions Every Woman Should Ask A Man

Laura Corn interviewed 1,000 men to find out what they really think about sex, love and relationships. These are the questions they most want to be asked by the women in their lives. Plus, men's outrageous, uncensored answers are sealed up inside.
($19.95 + $4.95 shipping & handling)

Audio Cassettes

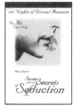

The Seven Secrets Of Seduction: For His Listening Pleasure Only!

The best of Laura's interviews and radio shows, specifically selected for men only. Sometimes hilarious, often shockingly erotic, always entertaining, this fast-paced tape features true confessions by men and women who have used Laura's Seven Secrets in their love lives. You won't believe your ears when you hear the reactions of America's most popular deejays! Two audio cassettes, 120 minutes.
($14.95 + $3.95 shipping & handling)

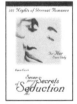

The Seven Secrets Of Seduction: For Her Listening Pleasure Only!

The best of Laura's interviews and radio shows, specifically selected for women only. Men and women from around the country talk frankly and explicitly about the impact Laura's Seven Secrets have had on their sexual relationships. Including some outrageous reactions by America's top-rated deejays, this tape is fast, funny, and full of astonishing insights by real lovers. Two audio cassettes, 120 minutes.
($14.95 + $3.95 shipping & handling)

To order your copies of any of these products,
or additional copies of *52 Invitations to Grrreat Sex* call:

1-800-547-2665

or send your check or money order to:
Park Avenue Publishers
903 S. Hohokam Drive.
Tempe, AZ 85281
(602) 829-0131

CA residents please 8.25% add sales tax

S P E C I A L T Y   S H O P S

For extensive catalogs including many of the
products mentioned in this book,
write or call the following companies:

For Adult Toys, Joys,
Videos, Books, Massage Oils, ETC:

Good Vibrations
1210 Valencia Street
San Francisco, Ca. 94110
1-800-289-8423

Eve's Garden
119 W. 57th Street
Suite 420
New York, NY 10019
212-575-8651
1-800-848-3837

For Flower Essences:

The Flower Essence Society
P.O. Box 459
Nevada City, Ca. 95959
800-548-0075

For Custom Blended Fragrance Oils:

Path of the Heart Fragrances
P.O. Box 3509
West Sedona, Az. 86340
928-282-9243